Alma-Ata 1978

Primary Health Care

Report of the

International Conference on Primary Health Care

Alma-Ata, USSR, 6-12 September 1978

Jointly sponsored by the World Health Organization
and the United Nations Children's Fund

WORLD HEALTH ORGANIZATION
GENEVA
1978

DECLARATION

The International Conference on Primary Health Care, meeting in Alma-Ata this twelfth day of September in the year Nineteen hundred and seventy-eight, expressing the need for urgent action by all governments, all health and development workers, and the world community to protect and promote the health of all the people of the world, hereby makes the following Declaration:

I

The Conference strongly reaffirms that health, which is a state of complete physical, mental and social wellbeing, and not merely the absence of disease or infirmity, is a fundamental human right and that the attainment of the highest possible level of health is a most important world-wide social goal whose realization requires the action of many other social and economic sectors in addition to the health sector.

II

The existing gross inequality in the health status of the people particularly between developed and developing countries as well as within countries is politically, socially and economically unacceptable and is, therefore, of common concern to all countries.

III

Economic and social development, based on a New International Economic Order, is of basic importance to the fullest attainment of health for all and to the reduction of the gap between the health status of the developing and developed countries. The promotion and pro-

OF ALMA-ATA

tection of the health of the people is essential to sustained economic and social development and contributes to a better quality of life and to world peace.

IV

The people have the right and duty to participate individually and collectively in the planning and implementation of their health care.

V

Governments have a responsibility for the health of their people which can be fulfilled only by the provision of adequate health and social measures. A main social target of governments, international organizations and the whole world community in the coming decades should be the attainment by all peoples of the world by the year 2000 of a level of health that will permit them to lead a socially and economically productive life. Primary health care is the key to attaining this target as part of development in the spirit of social justice.

VI

Primary health care is essential health care based on practical, scientifically sound and socially acceptable methods and technology made universally accessible to individuals and families in the community through their full participation and at a cost that the community and country can afford to maintain at every stage of their development in the spirit of self-reliance and self-determination. It forms an integral part both of the country's health system, of which it is the central function and main focus, and of the overall social and economic development of the community. It is the first level of contact of indi-

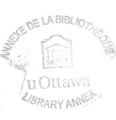

viduals, the family and community with the national health system bringing health care as close as possible to where people live and work, and constitutes the first element of a continuing health care process.

VII

Primary health care:

1. reflects and evolves from the economic conditions and socio-cultural and political characteristics of the country and its communities and is based on the application of the relevant results of social, biomedical and health services research and public health experience;

2. addresses the main health problems in the community, providing promotive, preventive, curative and rehabilitative services accordingly;

3. includes at least: education concerning prevailing health problems and the methods of preventing and controlling them; promotion of food supply and proper nutrition; an adequate supply of safe water and basic sanitation; maternal and child health care, including family planning; immunization against the major infectious diseases; prevention and control of locally endemic diseases; appropriate treatment of common diseases and injuries; and provision of essential drugs;

4. involves, in addition to the health sector, all related sectors and aspects of national and community development, in particular agriculture, animal husbandry, food, industry, education, housing, public works, communications and other sectors; and demands the coordinated efforts of all those sectors;

5. requires and promotes maximum community and individual self-reliance and participaton in the planning, organization, operation and control of primary health care, making fullest use of local, national and other available resources; and to this end develops through appropriate education the ability of communities to participate;

6. should be sustained by integrated, functional and mutually-supportive referral systems, leading to the progressive improvement of comprehensive health care for all, and giving priority to those most in need;

7. relies, at local and referral levels, on health workers, including physicians, nurses, midwives, auxiliaries and community workers as applicable, as well as traditional practitioners as needed, suitably trained socially and technically to work as a health team and to respond to the expressed health needs of the community.

VIII

All governments should formulate national policies, strategies and plans of action to launch and sustain primary health care as part of a comprehensive national health system and in coordination with other sectors. To this end, it will be necessary to exercise political will, to mobilize the country's resources and to use available external resources rationally.

IX

All countries should cooperate in a spirit of partnership and service to ensure primary health care for all people since the attainment of health by people in any one country directly concerns and benefits every other country. In this context the joint WHO/UNICEF report on primary health care constitutes a solid basis for the further development and operation of primary health care throughout the world.

X

An acceptable level of health for all the people of the world by the year 2000 can be attained through a fuller and better use of the world's resources, a considerable part of which is now spent on armaments and military conflicts. A genuine policy of independence, peace, détente and disarmament could and should release additional resources that could well be devoted to peaceful aims and in particular to the acceleration of social and economic development of which primary health care, as an essential part, should be allotted its proper share.

*　*　*

The International Conference on Primary Health Care calls for urgent and effective national and international action to develop and implement primary health care throughout the world and particularly in developing countries in a spirit of technical cooperation and in keeping with a New International Economic Order. It urges governments, WHO and UNICEF, and other international organizations, as well as multilateral and bilateral agencies, non-governmental organizations, funding agencies, all health workers and the whole world community to support national and international commitment to primary health care and to channel increased technical and financial support to it, particularly in developing countries. The Conference calls on all the aforementioned to collaborate in introducing, developing and maintaining primary health care in accordance with the spirit and content of this Declaration.

Contents

1. Background

1. As decided by the Health Assembly of the World Health Organization (WHO)[1] and the Executive Board of the United Nations Children's Fund (UNICEF), and at the invitation of the Government of the Union of Soviet Socialist Republics, the International Conference on Primary Health Care was held from 6 to 12 September 1978 in Alma-Ata, capital of the Kazakh Soviet Socialist Republic.

Introduction

2. The objectives of the Conference were:

Objectives

(i) to promote the concept of primary health care in all countries;

(ii) to exchange experience and information on the development of primary health care within the framework of comprehensive national health systems and services;

(iii) to evaluate the present health and health care situation throughout the world as it relates to, and can be improved by, primary health care;

(iv) to define the principles of primary health care as well as the operational means of overcoming practical problems in the development of primary health care;

(v) to define the role of governments, national, and international organizations in technical cooperation and support for the development of primary health care;

(vi) to formulate recommendations for the development of primary health care.

---

[1] Resolutions WHA28.88, adopted May 1975, and WHA29.19, adopted May 1976, which reaffirmed resolutions WHA20.53, WHA23.61, WHA25.17, WHA26.35, and WHA27.44 concerning the provision and promotion of effective comprehensive health care for all people and expressed the need to hold an international conference to exchange experience on the development of primary health care (WHO Handbook of Resolutions and Decisions, Vol. I, 1973, pp. 29, 30, 31 and Vol. II, (2nd ed.), 1977, pp. 19, 20, 21, 148).

3.   The International Conference on Primary Health Care, which was jointly organized and sponsored by the World Health Organization and the United Nations Children's Fund, was preceded by a number of national, regional, and international meetings on primary health care, held throughout the world in 1977 and 1978.   The regional and international meetings included: the meeting of the Committee of Experts on Primary Health Care in the African Region (Brazzaville, 1977), the Fourth Special Meeting of Ministers of Pan American Health Organization countries (Washington DC, September 1977), the Joint WHO/ UNICEF meeting for countries in the Eastern Mediterranean Region (Alexandria, October 1977), the Conference on Primary Health Care for countries in the Western Pacific Region (Manila, November 1977), the Joint WHO/UNICEF meeting on Primary Health Care in the South-East Asia Region (New Delhi, November 1977), the Conference on Primary Health Care in Industrialized Nations (New York, December 1977), and the International Congress of Nongovernmental Organizations on Primary Health Care (Halifax, Canada, May 1978).

4.   The documentation for the Conference consisted of a working paper, the joint report by the Director-General of WHO and the Executive Director of UNICEF entitled *Primary Health Care*,[1] and six regional background reports prepared by WHO Regional Directors, presenting different national experiences and approaches and a summary of critical issues to be faced at the national level.   In addition to this official Conference documentation, reports of national experiences and other materials, publications, examples of appropriate technology, photographs, and films related to primary health care were made available to the participants.   Participants also had the opportunity of visiting a number of exhibitions relating to primary health care including the health system in the USSR, organized by the host government, and appropriate technology for health, organized by UNICEF and the Kazakh SSR.

---

[1] See pages 35-79.

2. Attendance and Organization of Work

5.   The intergovernmental conference was attended by delegations from 134 governments and by representatives of 67 United Nations organizations, specialized agencies and nongovernmental organizations in official relations with WHO and UNICEF.

6.   Professor B. Petrovsky, Minister of Health of the USSR, was elected President of the Conference. The following were elected as Vice-Presidents of the Conference by acclamation: **Officers of the Conference**

> H.R.H. Princess Ashraf Pahlavi (Iran)
>
> Dr P. S. P. Dlamini (Swaziland)
>
> Dr Rodrigo Altman (Costa Rica)
>
> Sri J. Prasad Yadav (India)
>
> Dr Khamliene Pholsena (Lao People's Democratic Republic)

7.   The following were elected as Chairmen and Rapporteurs of the three main committees of the Conference:

Mr Jorge Chavez Quelopana (Peru)	Chairman, Committee A
Dr Manuel Rodriguei Boal (Guinea-Bissau)	Chairman, Committee B
Dr Kari Puro (Finland)	Chairman, Committee C
Professor W. A. Hassouna (Egypt)	Rapporteur, Committee A
Dr Francisco Aguilar (Philippines)	Rapporteur, Committee B
Professor Prapont Piyaratn (Thailand)	Rapporteur, Committee C

8.   The above-mentioned officers served as members of the General Committee together with those listed below:

> Professor E. Aujaleu (France)
>
> Mr Tsegaye Fekade (Ethiopia)
>
> Dr Abdul Rahman Kabbashi (Sudan)

Dr Roberto Lievano Perdomo (Colombia)

Miss Billie Miller (Barbados)

Mrs Antoinette Oliveira (Gabon)

Professor Georges Pinerd (Central African Empire)

Dr J. Bryant (deputizing for Dr Julius Richmond) (United States of America)

Mr E. Sanchez de León Perez (Spain)

Dr Siraj Ul-Haq Mahmud (Pakistan)

Professor K. Spies (German Democratic Republic)

Mr Mahess Teeluck (Mauritius)

Organization of work

9.   The Conference adopted an agenda and method of work, and agreed to divide major issues among three main committees: (i) Committee A to deal primarily with primary health care and development; (ii) Committee B to deal primarily with the technical and operational aspects of primary health care; (iii) Committee C to deal primarily with national strategies for primary health care and international support.

Addresses of welcome

10.   Addresses were delivered by Mr Kamaluddin Mohammed, President of the Thirty-first World Health Assembly, Professor J.J.A. Reid, Chairman of the WHO Executive Board, Dr Halfdan Mahler, Director-General of WHO, Mr Henry R. Labouisse, Executive Director of UNICEF, Dr T. Sh. Sharmanov, Minister of Health of the Kazakh SSR, on behalf of the host government, and Professor B. Petrovsky, President of the Conference.   Statements were made in plenary by government delegates and representatives of programmes and specialized agencies of the United Nations, liberation movements, and nongovernmental organizations.   It was proposed that addresses and statements on the theme of primary health care should be reproduced in a separate post-Conference document.

11.   Greetings were extended to all participants of the Conference by Mr D. A. Kunayev, member of the Presidium of the Supreme Soviet

of the USSR, who read out the text of the message of greetings from Mr L. I. Brezhnev, Secretary-General of the Communist Party and Chairman of the Presidium of the Supreme Soviet of the USSR.

12.   On 9-10 September 1978, the Conference participants were **Field visits** invited by the National Organizing Committee to visit different areas to acquaint themselves with the activities of health institutions in the cities and regions of Alma-Ata, Frunze, Karaganda, Chimkent, Tashkent, Samarkand, and Bukhara. They met with the Ministers of Health of the Kazakh, Kirghiz, and Uzbek union republics and other health service workers, visited feldscher and midwives' posts, rural and district hospitals, regional hospitals, emergency care services, sanitary and epidemiological stations, and other institutions. The organization and functions of these institutions were explained. The types of these institutions and the activities that they carry out have been changed periodically as required by the evolution of the health status of the population and the progressively developing capabilities of the health services, whereas the basic principles of the health system have remained the same. The plans for the further development of the health care system of the USSR were explained to the participants of the Conference during these visits.

3. Summary of Discussions

13. The Conference declared that the health status of hundreds of millions of people in the world today is unacceptable, particularly in developing countries. More than half the population of the world does not have the benefit of proper health care.

14. In view of the magnitude of health problems and the inadequate and inequitable distribution of health resources between and within countries, and believing that health is a fundamental human right and worldwide social goal, the Conference called for a new approach to health and health care, to close the gap between the "haves" and "have-nots", achieve more equitable distribution of health resources, and attain a level of health for all the citizens of the world that will permit them to lead a socially and economically productive life.

15. The Conference considered primary health care to be essential care based on practical, scientifically sound and socially acceptable methods and technology made universally accessible to individuals and families in the community through their full participation and at a cost that the community and country can afford to maintain at every stage of their development in the spirit of self-reliance and self-determination. It forms an integral part both of the country's health system, of which it is the central function and main focus, and of the overall social and economic development of the community. It is the first level of contact of individuals, the family, and the community with the national health system, bringing health care as close as possible to where people live and work, and constitutes the first element of a continuing health care process.

16. The Conference reaffirmed that governments have a responsibility for the health of their peoples which can be fulfilled only by

adequate and equitably distributed health and social measures. Primary health care, as part of the comprehensive national health care system, goes a long way to achieving these fundamental health and social objectives. Each country must interpret and adapt particular, detailed aspects of primary health care within the country's own social, political, and developmental context. All persons have the right and duty to participate individually and collectively in the planning and implementation of their health care.

17.   On the basis of experience in a number of countries, the Conference affirmed that the primary health care approach is essential to achieving an acceptable level of health throughout the world in the foreseeable future as an integral part of social development in the spirit of social justice. Thus the goal of thealth for all by the year 2000 would be attained.

18.   The Conference considered the close interrelationship and interdependence of health and social and economic development, with health leading to and at the same time depending on a progressive improvement in conditions and quality of life. The Conference stressed that primary health care is an integral part of the socioeconomic development process. Hence, activities of the health sector must be coordinated at national, intermediate, and community or local levels with those of other social and economic sectors, including education, agriculture, animal husbandry, household water, housing, public works, communications, and industry. Health activities should be undertaken concurrently with measures such as those for the improvement of nutrition, particularly of children and mothers; increase in production and employment, and a more equitable distribution of personal income; anti-poverty measures; and protection and improvement of the environment.

Primary health care and development

19.   The Conference emphasized the importance of full and organized community participation and ultimate self-reliance with individuals, families, and communities assuming more responsibility for their own

health. Community participation in the recognition and solution of their health problems can be facilitated by support from groups such as local government agencies, local leaders, voluntary groups, youth and women's groups, consumers' groups, the Red Cross and similar societies, other nongovernmental organizations, and liberation movements, as well as by accountability to the people. In order to ensure that primary health care is an integral part of community and national development and does not develop as an isolated peripheral action, promotion, co-ordination, and support of the administration are required, not only at the local but also at the intermediate and central levels.

20. The Conference affirmed the need for a balanced distribution of all available resources, and in particular government resources, so that appropriate attention is given to population groups deficient in terms of primary health care and overall development. National health development policies should give priority to making primary health care accessible to all as an integral part of a comprehensive health care system, taking into account geographical, social, cultural, political, economic, and other specific features of the country.

Technical and operational aspects

21. The Conference discussed the varied experience of countries in dealing with diverse health problems in rural and urban areas. It considered that ways of solving health problems vary from one country and community to another according to different stages of development, but should provide promotive, preventive, curative, rehabilitative, and emergency care appropriate to meet the main health problems in the community, with special attention to vulnerable groups, and be responsive to the needs and capacities of the people. The Conference reaffirmed the importance of establishing and further developing a comprehensive national health system of which primary health care is an integral part, encouraging the full participation of the population in all health-related activities.

22. It was stressed that all levels of the national health system have to support primary health care through appropriate training, super-

vision, referral, and logistic support. High priority should be given to the development of adequate manpower in health and related sectors, suitably trained for and attuned to primary health care, including traditional workers and traditional birth attendants, where appropriate. These workers should be organized to work as a team suited to the life-style and economic conditions of the country concerned.

23.   Primary health care requires the development, adaptation, and application of appropriate health technology that the people can use and afford, including an adequate supply of low-cost, good-quality essential drugs, vaccines, biologicals, and other supplies and equipment, as well as functionally efficient supportive health care facilities, such as health centres and hospitals. These facilities should be reoriented to the needs of primary health care and adapted to the socioeconomic environment.

24.   The Conference agreed that the translation of the principles of primary health care into action would require the priority allocation of budgetary resources to primary health care, better distribution and use of existing resources, and the improvement of managerial processes and capabilities at all levels for planning, implementing, budgeting, monitoring, supervising, and evaluating, supported by a relevant information system. Research with full involvement of populations in support of primary health care, especially health services research and the systematic application of knowledge in innovative ways, should be carried out to ensure that primary health care is included and progressively improved as an integral part, and main focus, of the comprehensive national health system. Development of indicators for planning, implementation, and evaluation of primary health care, including indicators for community participation and self-care, should be pursued.

25.   The Conference believed that, in adopting the Declaration of Alma-Ata, governments have made a historic collective expression of political will in the spirit of social equity aimed at improving health for all their peoples. Each nation should now make a strong and

National strategies and international support

19

continuing commitment to primary health care at all levels of government and society. Such a commitment should be clearly expressed as an integral part of the national health care system and other sectors of socioeconomic development. Governments should involve the people in this commitment.

26. It was stressed that national strategies are required to translate policies into action and to make health care available equitably to the entire population. National strategies should take into account socioeconomic factors and policies, available resources, and the particular health problems and needs of the population, with initial emphasis on the underserved. These strategies should be continuously reassessed in order to ensure their adaptation to evolving stages of development. The Conference emphasized that the strategies should be formulated and applied with the fullest possible participation of communities and all levels and sectors of government.

27. The Conference emphasized the multisectoral nature of health development and recognized that the success of any strategy for primary health care will require the full commitment and cooperation of all sectors of government. It further recognized that the improvement of health substantially contributes to increased productivity and wellbeing of the individual and the community. The Conference accordingly stressed the need for the health sector to take initiatives in ensuring that all factors affecting health receive the attention they deserve as well as working closely with the other sectors involved.

28. The Conference believed that countries can learn and benefit from each other's experience and urged all countries to cooperate among themselves in the promotion of primary health care through the sharing of information, experience, and expertise.

29. The Conference further believed that international organizations, multilateral and bilateral agencies, nongovernmental organizations, and other partners in international health should actively promote the national development of primary health care and give

increased technical and financial support with full respect for the principles of national self-reliance and self-determination and maximum utilization of locally available resources. Such organizations should provide information on available resources for technical cooperation. The Conference noted that any progress towards disarmament and the attainment of universal peace would release resources that could be used to accelerate socioeconomic development including primary health care, and also benefit populations suffering from the effects of armed conflict.

30. The Conference urged WHO and UNICEF to encourage and support national strategies and plans for primary health care as an essential part of overall development. They should also play a leading role in formulating concerted plans of action at the regional and global levels to facilitate the mutual support of countries and mobilize other international resources for accelerated development of primary health care.

31. The Conference expressed its deep appreciation and gratitude to the Governments and the people of the USSR and the Kazakh SSR for their excellent organization of the Conference and for the magnificent hospitality they extended to its participants. It also thanked the Governments and the people of the Kazakh SSR, the Uzbek SSR, and the Kirghiz SSR for the most interesting study tours of their health services that they organized for participants. The participants were impressed by the quality of these health services and wished them every success.

32. The Recommendations presented below and the Declaration of Alma-Ata were adopted by acclamation by the International Conference on Primary Health Care in plenary meeting on 12 September 1978.

33. During the closing ceremony one participant, indicated over-leaf, from each of WHO's six regions expressed the thanks of all par-

Closing ceremony

ticipants to the host country for the arrangements made on behalf of the International Conference on Primary Health Care:

Professor Rodrigo Altman	Costa Rica
Dr Abdoulaye Diallo	Mali
Professor Eugène Aujaleu	France
Dr A. A. Bukair	Democratic Yemen
Dr Raja Ahmad Noordin	Malaysia
Dr M. A. Matin	Bangladesh

34.   A farewell address by Dr T. H. Sharmanov, of the host country, was followed by a statement by Professor M. Petrovsky, President of the International Conference on Primary Health Care. The Conference closed with a formal reading of the Declaration of Alma-Ata by Dr Marcella Davies of Sierra Leone.

4. Recommendations

1. Interrelationships between health and development

The Conference,

Recognizing that health is dependent on social and economic development, and also contributes to it,

RECOMMENDS that governments incorporate and strengthen primary health care within their national development plans with special emphasis on rural and urban development programmes and the coordination of the health-related activities of the different sectors.

2. Community participation in primary health care

The Conference,

Considering that national and community self-reliance and social awareness are among the key factors in human development, and acknowledging that people have the right and duty to participate in the process for the improvement and maintenance of their health,

RECOMMENDS that governments encourage and ensure full community participation through the effective propagation of relevant information, increased literacy, and the development of the necessary institutional arrangements through which individuals, families, and communities can assume responsibility for their health and wellbeing.

3. The role of national administrations in primary health care

The Conference,

Noting the importance of appropriate administrative and financial support at all levels, for coordinated national development, including primary health care, and for translating national policies into practice,

RECOMMENDS that governments strengthen the support of their general administration to primary health care and related activities through coordination among different ministries and the delegation of appropriate responsibility and authority to intermediate and community levels, with the provision of sufficient manpower and resources to these levels.

4. Coordination of health and health-related sectors

The Conference,

Recognizing that significant improvement in the health of all people requires the planned and effective coordination of national health services and health-related activities of other sectors,

RECOMMENDS that national health policies and plans take full account of the inputs of other sectors bearing on health; that specific and workable arrangements be made at all levels—in particular at the intermediate and community levels—for the coordination of health services with all other activities contributing to health promotion and primary health care; and that arrangements for coordination take into account the role of the sectors dealing with administration and finance.

5. Content of primary health care

The Conference,

Stressing that primary health care should focus on the main health problems in the community, but recognizing that these problems and the ways of solving them will vary from one country and community to another,

RECOMMENDS that primary health care should include at least: education concerning prevailing health problems and the methods of identifying, preventing, and controlling them; promotion of food supply and proper nutrition, an adequate supply of safe water, and basic sanitation; maternal and child health care, including family planning; immunization against the major infectious diseases; prevention and control of locally endemic diseases; appropriate treatment of common diseases and injuries; promotion of mental health; and provision of essential drugs.

6. Comprehensive primary health care at the local level

The Conference,

Confirming that primary health care includes all activities that contribute to health at the interface between the community and the health system,

RECOMMENDS that, in order for primary health care to be comprehensive, all development-oriented activities should be interrelated and balanced so as to focus on problems of the highest priority as mutually perceived by the community and health system, and that culturally acceptable, technically appropriate, manageable, and appropriately selected interventions should be implemented in combinations that meet local needs. This implies that single-purpose programmes should be integrated into primary health care activities as quickly and smoothly as possible.

7. Support of primary health care within the national health system

The Conference,

Considering that primary health care is the foundation of a comprehensive national health system and that the health system must be organized to support primary health care and make it effective,

RECOMMENDS that governments promote primary health care and related development activities so as to enhance the capacity and determination of the people to solve their own problems. This requires a close relationship between the primary health care workers and the community and that each team be responsible for a defined area. It also necessitates reorienting the existing system to ensure that all levels of the health system support primary health care by facilitating referral of patients and consultation on health problems; by providing supportive supervision and guidance, logistic support, and supplies; and through improved use of referral hospitals.

8. Special needs of vulnerable and high-risk groups

The Conference,

Recognizing the special needs of those who are least able, for geographical, political, social, or financial reasons, to take the initiative in seeking health care, and expressing great concern for those who are the most vulnerable or at greatest risk,

RECOMMENDS that, as part of total coverage of populations through primary health care, high priority be given to the special needs of women, children, working populations at high risk, and the underprivileged segments of society, and that the necessary activities be maintained, reaching out into all homes and working places to identify systematically those at highest risk, to provide continuing care to them, and to eliminate factors contributing to ill healh.

9. Roles and categories of health and health-related manpower for primary health care

The Conference,

Recognizing that the development of primary health care depends on the attitudes and capabilities of all health workers and also on a health system that is designed to support and complement the frontline workers,

RECOMMENDS that governments give high priority to the full utilization of human resources by defining the technical role, supportive skills, and attitudes required for each category of health worker according to the functions that need to be carried out to ensure effective primary health care, and by developing teams composed of community health workers, other developmental workers, intermediate personnel, nurses, midwives, physicians, and, where applicable, traditional practitioners and traditional birth attendants.

10. Training of health and health-related manpower for primary health care

The Conference,

Recognizing the need for sufficient numbers of trained personnel for the support and delivery of primary health care,

RECOMMENDS that governments undertake or support reorientation and training for all levels of existing personnel and revised programmes for the training of new community health personnel; that health workers, especially physicians and nurses, should be socially and technically trained and motivated to serve the community; that all training should include field activities; that physicians and other professional health workers should be urged to work in underserved areas early in their career; and that due attention should be paid to continuing education, supportive supervision, the preparation of teachers of health workers, and health training for workers from other sectors.

11. Incentives for service in remote and neglected areas

The Conference,

Recognizing that service in primary health care focused on the needs of the underserved requires special dedication and motivation, but that even then there is a crucial need to provide culturally suitable rewards and recognition for service under difficult and rigorous conditions,

RECOMMENDS that all levels of health personnel be provided with incentives scaled to the relative isolation and difficulty of the conditions under which they live and work. These incentives should be adapted to local situations and may take such forms as better living and working conditions and opportunities for further training and continuing education.

12. Appropriate technology for health

The Conference,

Recognizing that primary health care requires the identification, development, adaptation, and implementation of appropriate technology,

RECOMMENDS that governments, research and academic institutions, nongovernmental organizations, and especially communities, develop technologies and methods that contribute to health, both in the health system and in associated services; are scientifically sound, adapted to local needs, and acceptable to the community; and are maintained by the people themselves, in keeping with the principle of self-reliance, with resources the community and the country can afford.

13. Logistic support and facilities for primary health care

The Conference,

Aware that the success of primary health care depends on adequate, appropriate, and sustained logistic support in thousands of communities in many countries, raising new problems of great magnitude,

RECOMMENDS that governments ensure that efficient administrative, delivery, and maintenance services be established, reaching out to all primary health care activities at the community level; that suitable and sufficient supplies and equipment be always available at all levels in the health system, in particular to community health workers; that careful attention be paid to the safe delivery and storage of perishable supplies such as vaccines; that there be appropriate strengthening of support facilities including hospitals, and that governments ensure that transport and all physical facilities for primary health care be functionally efficient and appropriate to the social and economic environment.

14. Essential drugs for primary health care

The Conference,

Recognizing that primary health care requires a continuous supply of essential drugs; that the provision of drugs accounts for a significant proportion of expenditures in the health sector; and that the progressive extension of primary health care to ensure eventual national coverage entails a large increase in the provision of drugs,

RECOMMENDS that governments formulate national policies and regulations with respect to the import, local production, sale, and distribution of drugs and biologicals so as to ensure that essential drugs are available at the various levels of primary health care at the lowest feasible cost; that specific measures be taken to prevent the over utilization of medicines; that proved traditional remedies be incorporated; and that effective administrative and supply systems be established.

15. Administration and management for primary health care

The Conference,

Considering that the translation of the principles of primary health care into practice requires the strengthening of the administrative structure and managerial processes,

RECOMMENDS that governments should develop the administrative framework and apply at all levels appropriate managerial processes to plan for and implement primary health care, improve the allocation and distribution of resources, monitor and evaluate programmes with the help of a simple and relevant information system, share control with the community, and provide appropriate management training of health workers of different categories.

16. Health services research and operational studies

The Conference,

Emphasizing that enough is known about primary health care for governments to initiate or expand its implementation, but also recognizing that many long-range and complex issues need to be resolved, that the contribution of traditional systems of medicine calls for further research, and that new problems are constantly emerging as implementation proceeds,

RECOMMENDS that every national programme should set aside a percentage of its funds for continuing health services research; organize health services research and development units and field areas that operate in parallel with the general implementation process; encourage evaluation and feedback for early identification of problems; give responsibility to educational and research institutions and thus bring them into close collaboration with the health system; encourage the involvement of field workers and community members; and undertake a sustained effort to train research workers in order to promote national self-reliance.

17. Resources for primary health care

The Conference,

Recognizing that the implementation of primary health care requires the effective mobilization of resources bearing on health,

RECOMMENDS that, as an expression of their political determination to promote the primary health care approach, governments, in progressively increasing the funds allocated for health, should give first priority to the extension of primary health care to underserved communities; encourage and support various ways of financing primary health care, including, where appropriate, such means as social insurance, cooperatives, and all available resources at the local level, through the active involvement and participation of communities; and take measures to maximize the efficiency and effectiveness of health-related activities in all sectors.

18. National commitment to primary health care

The Conference,

Affirming that primary health care requires strong and continued political commitment at all levels of government, based upon the full understanding and support of the people,

RECOMMENDS that governments express their political will to attain health for all by making a continuing commitment to implement primary health care as an integral part of the national health system within overall socioeconomic development, with the involvement of all sectors concerned; to adopt enabling legislation where necessary; and to stimulate, mobilize, and sustain public interest and participation in the development of primary health care.

19. National strategies for primary health care

The Conference,

Stressing the need for national strategies to translate policies for primary health care into action,

RECOMMENDS that governments elaborate without delay national strategies with well-defined goals and develop and implement plans of action to ensure that primary health care be made accessible to the entire population, the highest priority being given to underserved areas and groups, and reassess these policies, strategies, and plans for primary health care, in order to ensure their adaptation to evolving stages of development.

20. Technical cooperation in primary health care

The Conference,

Recognizing that all countries can learn from each other in matters of health and development,

RECOMMENDS that countries share and exchange information, experience, and expertise in the development of primary health care as part of technical cooperation among countries, particularly among developing countries.

21. International support for primary health care

The Conference,

Realizing that in order to promote and sustain health care and overcome obstacles to its implementation there is a need for strong, coordinated, international solidarity and support, and
Welcoming the offers of collaboration from United Nations organizations as well as from other sources of cooperation,

RECOMMENDS that international organizations, multilateral and bilateral agencies, nongovernmental organizations, funding agencies, and other partners in international health acting in a coordinated manner should encourage and support national commitment to primary health care and should channel increased technical and financial support into it, with full respect for the coordination of these resources by the countries themselves in a spirit of self-reliance and self-determination, as well as with the maximum utilization of locally available resources.

22. Role of WHO and UNICEF in supporting primary health care

The Conference,

Recognizing the need for a world plan of action for primary health care as a cooperative effort of all countries,

RECOMMENDS that WHO and UNICEF, guided by the declaration of Alma-Ata and the recommendations of this Conference, should continue to encourage and support national strategies and plans for primary health care as part of overall development.

RECOMMENDS that WHO and UNICEF, on the basis of national strategies and plans, formulate as soon as possible concerted plans of action at the regional and global levels that promote and facilitate the mutual support of countries, particularly through the use of their national institutions, for accelerated development of primary health care.

RECOMMENDS that WHO and UNICEF continuously promote the mobilization of other international resources for primary health care.

Primary Health Care

A joint report by

The Director-General of the World Health Organization

and

The Executive Director of the United Nations Children's Fund

presented at the

International Conference on Primary Health Care

Alma-Ata, USSR, 6-12 September 1978

PRIMARY

Primary Health Care is essential health care made universally accessible to individuals and families in the community by means acceptable to them, through their full participation and at a cost that the community and country can afford. It forms an integral part both of the country's health system of which it is the nucleus and of the overall social and economic development of the community.

Primary Health Care addresses the main health problems in the community, providing promotive, preventive, curative and rehabilitative services accordingly. Since these services reflect and evolve from the economic conditions and social values of the country and its communities, they will vary by country and community, but will include at least: promotion of proper nutrition and an adequate supply of safe water; basic sanitation; maternal and child care, including family planning; immunization against the major infectious diseases; prevention and control of locally endemic diseases; education concerning prevailing health problems and the methods of preventing and controlling them; and appropriate treatment for common diseases and injuries.

In order to make Primary Health Care universally accessible in the community as quickly as possible, maximum community and individual self-reliance for health development are essential. To attain such self-reliance requires full community participation in the planning, organization and management of Primary Health Care. Such partici-

HEALTH CARE

pation is best mobilized through appropriate education which enables communities to deal with their real health problems in the most suitable ways. They will thus be in a better position to take rational decisions concerning Primary Health Care and to make sure that the right kind of support is provided by the other levels of the national health system. These other levels have to be organized and strengthened so as to support Primary Health Care with technical knowledge, training, guidance and supervision, logistic support, supplies, information, financing and referral facilities including institutions to which unsolved problems and individual patients can be referred.

Primary Health Care is likely to be most effective if it employs means that are understood and accepted by the community and applied by community health workers at a cost the community and the country can afford. These community health workers, including traditional practitioners where applicable, will function best if they reside in the community they serve and are properly trained socially and technically to respond to its expressed health needs.

Since Primary Health Care is an integral part both of the country's health system and of overall economic and social development, without which it is bound to fail, it has to be coordinated on a national basis with the other levels of the health system as well as with the other sectors that contribute to a country's total development strategy.

1. General Outline

1. Primary health care is the key to achieving an acceptable level of health throughout the world in the foreseeable future as part of social development and in the spirit of social justice. It is equally valid for all countries, from the most to the least developed, though the form it takes will vary according to political, economic, social and cultural patterns. For developing countries in particular, it is a burning necessity. For this reason, this report will concentrate on the needs of these countries. **Introduction**

2. The gap is widening between the health "haves" in the affluent countries and the health "have-nots" in the developing world. Moreover, this gap is also evident within individual countries, whatever their level of development. **The situation now**

3. There is widespread disenchantment with health care throughout the world. The reasons are not difficult to discern. Better health could be achieved with the technical knowledge available. Unfortunately, in most countries this knowledge is not being put to the best advantage for the greatest number. Health resources are allocated mainly to sophisticated medical institutions in urban areas. Quite apart from the dubious social premise on which this is based, the concentration of complex and costly technology on limited segments of the population does not even have the advantage of improving health. Indeed, the improvement of health is being equated with the provision of medical care dispensed by growing numbers of specialists, using narrow medical technologies for the benefit of the privileged few. People have have become cases without personalities, and contact has been lost between those providing medical care and those receiving it.

4. At the same time, disadvantaged groups throughout the world have no access to any permanent form of health care. These groups

probably total four-fifths of the world's population, living mainly in rural areas and urban slums. In some countries, even though health facilities are located within easy reach, inability to pay or cultural taboos put them out of bounds.

5. To complicate matters, health systems are all too often being devised outside the mainstream of social and economic development. These systems frequently restrict themselves to medical care, although industrialization and deliberate alteration of the environment are creating health problems whose proper control lies far beyond the scope of medical care.

6. Thus, most conventional health care systems are becoming increasingly complex and costly and have doubtful social relevance. They have been distorted by the dictates of medical technology and by the misguided efforts of a medical industry providing medical consumer goods to society. Even some of the most affluent countries have come to realize the disparity between the high care costs and low health benefits of these systems. Obviously it is out of the question for the developing countries to continue importing them. Other approaches have to be sought.

The primary health care approach

7. Primary health care is a practical approach to making essential health care universally accessible to individuals and families in the community in an acceptable and affordable way and with their full participation. This approach has evolved over the years, partly in the light of experience, positive and negative, gained in basic health services in a number of countries. But it means much more than the mere extension of basic health services. It has social and developmental dimensions and if properly applied will influence the way in which the rest of the health system functions.

8. Its shape is determined by social goals, such as the improvment of the quality of life and maximum health benefits to the greatest number; and these goals are attained by social means, such as the

acceptance of greater responsibility for health by communities and individuals and their active participation in attaining it. The healthier people are, the more likely they are to be able to contribute to social and economic development, and such development in turn provides the additional resources and social energy that can facilitate health development. So primary health care and community efforts towards social and economic development in general are most likely to succeed when they are mutually supportive. Also, just as the health sector functions best in harmony with the other social and economic sectors, so there is a need for harmony within the health sector through support to primary health care by all other levels.

9. The time has come for all levels of the health system to review critically their methods, techniques, equipment and drugs, with the aim of using only those technologies that have really proved their worth and can be afforded. For primary health care this is vital, because there has been a tendency to concentrate on medical technologies that are more appropriate for hospital use than for front-line care. The scope and purpose of primary health care, and the technical capacity of those who provide it, make it more important than ever to have appropriate technology available.

10. Primary health care is delivered by community health workers. The skills these workers require, and therefore their training, will vary widely throughout the world, depending upon the particular form of primary health care being provided. Whatever their level of skill, it is important that they understand the real health needs of the communities they serve, and that they gain the confidence of the people. This implies that they should reside in the community they are serving, and in many societies that they should be chosen by it.

Health system support

11. The support of other levels of the health system is necessary to ensure that people enjoy the benefits of valid and useful technical knowledge that is too complex or costly to apply routinely through primary health care. These levels are an important source of relevant

information on health. Moreover, community health workers must be able to rely on more skilled people for guidance and training, and primary health care services need the security of logistic and financial support.

12. The acceptance of primary health care therefore implies the organization of the rest of the health system so as to provide support for primary health care and to enhance its further development. This means that the health system as a whole will have to accept the social goal of making essential health care available to all. The consequence for health policy is the preferential allocation of resources to people at the social periphery in order to satisfy first and foremost their essential health care needs, for experience has shown that overall improvements in national health situations depend on improving the health status of these people. Fortified by additional resources, communities will be in a better position to accept greater responsibility for their own health, and to fulfil this responsibility through primary health care. The more specialized needs of this care will influence the type of service that has to be provided by the more central levels of the health system. The result should be stronger links between the more centrally placed health institutions and the communities they are intended to serve.

Coordination with other sectors

13. Health cannot be attained by the health sector alone. In developing countries in particular, economic development, anti-poverty measures, food production, water, sanitation, housing, environmental protection and education all contribute to health and have the same goal of human development. Primary health care, as an integral part of the health system and of overall social and economic development, will of necessity rest on proper coordination at all levels between the health and all other sectors concerned.

Improvement through learning and research

14. The principles of primary health care are known, but they are undoubtedly capable of progressive improvement and extension. In practice, many different forms exist throughout the world, and lessons

can be learned from all of them. For example, it would be useful to know more about community participation and behaviour, joint action with other sectors, appropriate technology, training and supervision of community health workers and questions relating to their careers, means of support and referral, and methods of communication between primary health care and other levels of the health system. Much can be learned by doing, but in addition there is a need for organized research that is closely linked to the provision of service.

15. It can be seen that the proper application of primary health care will have far-reaching consequences, not only throughout the health sector but also for other social and economic sectors at the community level. Moreover, it will greatly influence community organization in general. Resistance to such change is only to be expected; for instance, attempts to ensure a more equitable distribution of health resources could well meet with resistance from political and professional pressure groups, and the use of appropriate technology may arouse the opposition of the medical industries.

Ways of overcoming obstacles

16. Obstacles such as these can be overcome if they are prepared for in advance. The most important single factor in promoting primary health care and overcoming obstacles is a strong political will and support at both national and community level, reinforced by a firm national strategy. But specific antidotes can also be employed. For example, it may be possible to influence those health professionals not already convinced of the importance of primary health care by involving them in its development. They will need to be persuaded that they are not relinquishing medical functions but gaining health responsibilities. In the same way, resistance among the general public can be defused by discussions in communities and in the mass media. These discussions should aim to make people appreciate that primary health care is realistic, since it provides, at a cost that can be afforded, essential health care for all in a spirit of social justice rather than sophisticated medical care for the few in a counter spirit of social inequality.

17.   Opposition from the medical industries can be directed into positive channels by interesting them in the production of equipment for appropriate technology to be used in primary health care. Any losses from reduced sales of limited amounts of expensive equipment could well be more than counterbalanced by the sale to large untapped markets of greater amounts of less expensive equipment and supplies for primary health care.

18.   Reservations may be voiced by certain schools of economic planning, based on the common belief that economic growth alone will bring in its wake the solution of health problems. In answer to this it should be explained that, whereas real social and economic development can undoubtedly bring about improvements in health, there is also a need to apply direct health measures to improve health situations and that, as mentioned above, efforts from all the sectors concerned are mutually supportive.

19.   There may even be misguided support for primary health care based on the wrong assumption that it implies the cheapest form of medical care for the poor, with the bare minimum of financial and technical support. Only political intervention, coupled with forceful explanations of the real purpose and scope of primary health care, can overcome such an attitude.

Political and financial implications

20.   Political commitment to primary health care implies more than formal support from the government and community leaders. It requires the reorientation of national health development strategies. For developing countries in particular, it implies the transfer of a greater share of health resources to the underserved majority of the population. At the same time, there is a need to increase the national health budget until the total population has access to essential health care. Much of this increase will have to be devoted to those institutions providing direct support to primary health care.

21. The implications of political commitment by the developed countries to primary health care are equally far-reaching and, moreover, have a direct bearing on the efforts of the developing countries. Developed countries, too, need to rationalize their health care systems and stem their rising costs. Also, an explicit policy is required whereby the affluent countries commit themselves to a more equitable distribution of international health resources to enable the developing countries, and especially the least developed, to apply primary health care.

22. International governmental and nongovernmental agencies should now be encouraged to give priority attention within the health field to primary health care. Furthermore, the adoption of a global primary health care policy and strategy will be extremely important to support national policies and strategies and their proper implementation. **Need for global action**

23. The time has come for primary health care to be firmly implanted in the world political scene. This requires international agreement on the adoption of a worldwide primary health care policy and strategy with the goal of making essential health care available to all the people of the world. It also requires international action to ensure the unstinting support of the international community, and to encourage countries to set primary health care in motion, to maintain its momentum, and to cooperate in overcoming obstacles. The display of such international determination will provide an outstanding illustration of the practical application of technical cooperation among countries, whatever their level of development.

2. Primary Health Care and Development

Interrelationships between health and development

24. Development implies progressive improvements in the living conditions and quality of life enjoyed by society and shared by its members. It is a continuing process that takes place in all societies; few would claim that their development is complete.

25. Any distinction between economic and social development is no longer tenable. Economic development is necessary to achieve most social goals and social development is necessary to achieve most economic goals. Indeed, social factors are the real driving force behind development. The purpose of development is to permit people to lead economically productive and socially satisfying lives. Social satisfaction and economic productivity will be interpreted in widely different ways according to the social and cultural values prevailing in each society. Everywhere people themselves realize that their motivation in striving to increase their earnings is not greater wealth for its own sake but the social improvements that increased purchasing power can bring to them and their children, such as better food and housing, better education, better leisure opportunities, and, last but not least, better health. Only when they have an acceptable level of health can individuals, families and communities enjoy the other benefits of life. Health development is therefore essential for social and economic development, and the means for attaining them are intimately linked. For this reason, actions to improve the health and socioeconomic situation should be regarded as mutually supportive rather than competitive. Discussions on whether the promotion of health only consumes resources, or whether it is an economically productive factor contributing to development, belong to the academic past.

44

26. Since primary health care is the key to attaining an acceptable level of health by all, it will help people to contribute to their own social and economic development. It follows that primary health care should be an integral part of the overall development of society.

Contribution of primary health care to development

27. Primary health care contributes to development by improving health status and by stimulating action and organization in support of the development process. As an example, the control of certain communicable diseases by primary health care and other means often helps to promote development in general. For instance, the control of malaria, sleeping sickness and river blindness can open new areas to settlement, but these successes have to be consolidated by maintaining the settlers' health and their potential for development. Proper nutrition and reduction of sickness increase work productivity. Breaking the vicious circle of malnutrition and infection improves the physical and mental development of the child. In societies where old people are cared for directly by their family, a reduction in infant mortality can eventually lead to a reduction in family size, because the continued existence and health of the first two or three children provide couples with the security they are seeking for their old age. In general, a reduction in both child and adult mortality can induce the feeling that the future is worth planning for. In addition, by drawing on untapped human and financial community resources, primary health care can contribute to the awakening of the social interest that is so important for mobilizing people's efforts for development. Thus, primary health care can be a lever for increasing social awareness and interest, initiative and innovation.

28. The other levels of the country's health system can also assist development on condition that they are attuned to providing support to the full range of primary health care activities. For example, they can concentrate selectively on combating health risks which directly or indirectly influence poverty. In addition to providing specialized curative services, they can catalyse development by supporting community activities that promote health and prevent disease. They can play a wider role in the training of health workers by showing them

how to function in harmony with workers in related social and economic fields for the common purpose of development. They can help to ensure the acceptance, at the appropriate administrative levels, of ideas and proposals emanating from communities that will promote an integrated approach to health and development. They can also help to shape, at these administrative levels, the mechanisms for arriving at decisions that are conducive to integrated development.

Support to primary health care from other sectors

29. No sector involved in socioeconomic development can function properly in isolation. Activities in one impinge on the goals of another; hence the need for constant consultation between the major social and economic sectors to ensure development and to promote health as part of it. Primary health care, too, requires the support of other sectors; these sectors can also serve as entry points for the development and implementation of primary health care.

30. The *agricultural sector* is particularly important in most countries. It can ensure that production of food for family consumption becomes an integral part of agricultural policy and that food actually reaches those who produce it, which in some countries may require changes in the pattern of land tenure. Also, nutritional status can be improved through programmes in agriculture and home economics geared to meeting priority family and community needs.

31. It is particularly important to ensure that *women* enjoy the benefits of agricultural development as well as men. In most developing countries the majority of women in rural areas are engaged simultaneously in agriculture, household management and the care of infants and children. They need appropriate technology to lighten their workload and increase their work productivity. They also require knowledge about nutrition which they can apply with the resources available, in particular concerning the proper feeding of children and their own nutrition during pregnancy and lactation.

32.   Similar policies in support of health are needed in other sectors. *Water* for household use is as important as water for cattle, irrigation, energy and industry.   Plentiful supplies of clean water help to decrease mortality and morbidity, in particular among infants and children, as well as making life easier for women.   Countrywide plans are required to bring urban and rural water supplies within easy reach of the majority in the shortest possible time.   This is in keeping with the target adopted by Habitat, the United Nations Conference on Human Settlements, of having safe water for all by the year 1990.   The safe disposal of wastes and excreta also has a significant influence on health.

33.   The health sector can promote investments in water supply and sanitation, but as a rule major investments come from other sectors.   In rural areas in particular, the community may well be active in these fields as part of primary health care.   Education in the proper use and maintenance of water and sanitary facilities is important.

34.   *Housing* that is properly adapted to local climatic and environmental conditions has a positive effect on health.   Houses, like animal shelters and food storage facilities, need to be proof not only against the elements but also against insects and rodents that carry disease. All these structures, and particularly kitchens and sanitary facilities, should be easy to clean.   Here too, education is important for ensuring the proper maintenance of houses and the areas surrounding them.

35.   Certain aspects of *public works and communications* are of strategic importance to primary health care, particularly for dispersed populations.   Feeder roads not only connect the farmer to the market but also make it easier for people to reach villages, bringing new ideas together with the supplies needed for health and other sectors.   Two-way radio communication, where this can be afforded, puts isolated areas in contact with more centrally located administrative levels, at the same time serving as a vehicle for learning.   Low-cost pedal-operated radio communication has been successfully used in primary health care in a number of developing countries.

36.   The *educational sector* also has an important part to play in the development and operation of primary health care. Community education helps people to understand their health problems, possible solutions to them and the cost of different alternatives. Instructive literature can be developed and distributed through the educational system. Associations of parents and teachers can assume certain responsibilities for primary health care activities within schools and the community, such as sanitation programmes, food-for-health campaigns or courses on nutrition and first aid.

37.   The *mass media* can play a supportive educational role by providing valid information on health and ways of attaining it and by depicting the benefits to be derived from improved health practices within primary health care. For example, they could support a sound pharmaceutical policy by helping to create public awareness that a number of drugs with generic names are just as good as advertised products with brand names. They could also help to popularize primary health care by disseminating authentic news about it in different communities.

38.   Many *agricultural and industrial activities* can have side effects that are detrimental to health. To mention a few, irrigation schemes can create the right conditions for the breeding of mosquitos that transmit malaria, artificial lakes can lead to the proliferation of the snails that carry schistosomiasis, industrialization can lead to the pollution of air and water with toxic chemicals and the accompanying urbanization can provoke psychosocial problems. It is therefore wise to incorporate preventive measures in industrial and agricultural projects which pose particular health hazards. Such measures can be included in irrigation schemes and man-made lakes, safety precautions can be taken to reduce industrial accidents and pollution, potential carriers of disease can be identified wherever there are large population movements, and special attention can be given to protecting the physical and mental health of migrant workers. There is a proper place for primary health care in most of these activities.

39. In addition, the industrial sector can support primary health care by establishing industries related to health, in particular for essential foods and drugs. Local small-scale industries are also important, because they create employment and thereby improve the local economic base and earning power.

40. Coordinated planning at the community level will make it possible to link primary health care closely with other sectors in joint efforts for community development. Thus, community workers can be trained to provide services of different kinds and to complement one another's roles. For example, the health worker can advise on the importance of improved food storage at home and on the farm and can give practical guidance on this matter. Similarly, the agricultural worker who understands the basic principles of good nutrition can influence the production of appropriate foods and their consumption by families, helped by a local agricultural policy that favours food crops rather than cash crops.

Coordination of development activities at the community level

41. Community representatives in local government can ensure that community interests are properly taken into account in the planning and implementation of development programmes. Of overriding importance is the principle that public services should be accountable to the communities they serve, in particular for resources that the latter have invested. The desirability of coordinating at the local level the activities of the various sectors involved in socioeconomic development, and the crucial role of the community in achieving this integration, make community participation an essential component of primary health care.

42. A community consists of people living together in some form of social organization and cohesion. Its members share in varying degrees political, economic, social and cultural characteristics, as well as interests and aspirations, including health. Communities vary widely

Community participation

in size and socioeconomic profile, ranging from clusters of isolated homesteads to more organized villages, towns and city districts.

43.   Self-reliance and social awareness are key factors in human development. Community participation in deciding on policies and in planning, implementing and controlling development programmes is now a widely accepted practice. However, it is understood and interpreted in different ways in different countries, being greatly influenced by the overall political structure and the social and economic situation. The case studies on community participation conducted by the UNICEF/ WHO Joint Committee on Health Policy have helped to draw attention to and clarify the role of community participation in primary health care.

44.   Community participation is the process by which individuals and families assume responsibility for their own health and welfare and for those of the community, and develop the capacity to contribute to their and the community's development. They come to know their own situation better and are motivated to solve their common problems. This enables them to become agents of their own development instead of passive beneficiaries of development aid. They therefore need to realize that they are not obliged to accept conventional solutions that are unsuitable but can improvise and innovate to find solutions that are suitable. They have to acquire the capacity to appraise a situation, weigh the various possibilities and estimate what their own contribution can be. While the community must be willing to learn, the health system is responsible for explaining and advising, and for providing clear information about the favourable and adverse consequences of the interventions being proposed, as well as their relative costs.

45.   Health personnel form part of the community in which they live and work. A continuing dialogue between them and the rest of the community is necessary to harmonize views and activities relating to primary health care. Such a dialogue enables health personnel to acquire a better understanding of the community's feelings, the reasons

for its views, the level of its aspirations and the pattern of its organization and communications. For their part, the people will learn to identify their real health needs, to understand the national strategy for primary health care and to become involved in and promote community action for health. Thus, society will come to realize that health is not only the right of all but also the responsibility of all, and the members of the health professions, too, will find their proper role.

46.   There are many ways in which the community can participate in every stage of primary health care. It must first be involved in the assessment of the situation, the definition of problems and the setting of priorities. Then, it helps to plan primary health care activities and subsequently it cooperates fully when these activities are carried out. Such cooperation includes the acceptance by individuals of a high degree of responsibility for their own health care—for example, by adopting a healthy life style, by applying principles of good nutrition and hygiene, or by making use of immunization services. In addition, members of the community can contribute labour as well as financial and other resources to primary health care.

47.   It is also a proper community concern to keep the implementation of primary health care under constant review and to make sure that it functions in accordance with its stated purpose. This involvement will facilitate the identification and resolution of difficulties and the readjustment of activities as necessary.

48.   A clear national policy is needed which will promote community cohesion around efforts for health and related development, will foster the coordination at the local level of all sectoral programmes that have a bearing on primary health care, will build up the capacity of communities to make their health and other social aspirations known, and will ensure that the community controls both the funds it invests in primary health care and the personnel providing it. Community participation also requires mutual support between government and community, reinforced by mutual information feedback. It is the responsibility of government to stimulate this kind of support, to set

up the necessary intersectoral coordinating mechanisms at the different administrative levels, to pass legislation to support primary health care and, wherever applicable, to provide sufficient human, material, technical and financial resources.

Decentralization in the development process

49.   The general administrative system of a country is important for ensuring coordinated contributions to development from the different sectors concerned.   In the past, these has been a tendency to concentrate almost entirely on the central administrative level.   Only recently has attention been focused on local levels.   The importance of decentralization to intermediate levels, such as provincial or district levels, now has to be stressed.   These levels are near enough to communities to respond sensitively to their practical problems and needs;   they are equally near to the central administrative level to translate government policies into practice.   They are particularly useful for harmonizing the activities of the various sectors that jointly promote development.   The intermediate administrative levels thus serve as important pivots for coordinated development.   To fulfil this role they have to be strengthened in many countries, particularly by deploying to them the manpower required in the various sectors.

3. Operational Aspects of Primary Health Care

50.   A health system is made up of components from the health and other sectors whose interrelated actions contribute to health.   It is subdivided into various levels, the first of which is the point of contact between individuals and the health system, where primary health care is delivered.   The services provided by primary health care will vary according to the country and the community, but will include at least: promotion of proper nutrition and an adequate supply of safe water; basic sanitation;   maternal and child care, including family planning; immunization against the major infectious diseases;   prevention and control of locally endemic diseases; education concerning prevailing health problems and the methods of preventing and controlling them; and appropriate treatment for common diseases and injuries.   The other levels of the health system provide more specialized services which become more complex as they become more central.

Primary health care within the health system

51.   Primary health care is the hub of the health system.   Around it are arranged the other levels of the system whose actions converge on primary health care in order to support it and to permit it to provide essential health care on a continuing basis.   At the intermediate level more complex problems can be dealt with, and more skilled and specialized care as well as logistic support provided.   At this level, more highly trained staff provide support through training and through guidance on practical problems that arise in connexion with all aspects of primary health care.   The central level provides planning and managerial expertise, highly specialized care, teaching for specialist staff, the expertise of such institutions as central health laboratories, and central logistic and financial support.   How the health system is organized to develop, operate and support primary health care is the subject of the following paragraphs.

Planning   52.   Planning for primary health care has to be carried out in communities as well as at intermediate and central levels. The ministry of health or its equivalent is responsible for formulating national health policy, including primary health care policy, and for promoting its adoption by the government. Such policies are more likely to be effective if they form part of overall development policies, thus reflecting the social and economic goals of the government. Strategies have to be devised to translate policies into practice; a useful process for this purpose has come to be known as *country health programming*, which consists essentially of assessing the country's health problems in their socioeconomic context, identifying areas susceptible to change and formulating priority programmes to induce such change.

53.   Wherever primary health care has been identified as a priority, which is likely to be the case in most countries, a specific strategy is needed for its formulation and implementation. The primary health care policy and strategy form the terms of reference for all the health and relevant components of other sectors which make up the health system. The strategy has to be translated into a nationwide primary health care programme embracing all levels, supportive and referral as well as community.

54.   In developing the strategy and formulating the programme, full account has to be taken of the technologies to be used, the resources to be employed, the support needed at other levels, and the way to organize all this into a coherent system.

55.   Health ministries, as well as other national health agencies that may be concerned, need to make planning a function of the highest level of decision-making. This is essential to ensure the appropriate delegation of responsibility and authority, the preferential allocation of resources to primary health care and its supporting services, and the proper location of the supporting services so that they are accessible to the communities they are to serve. Training in planning and management at all levels is indispensable to the planning process. Since the

planning of primary health care involves political, social and economic factors, multidisciplinary planning teams are needed, especially at the central level, including among others people with a knowledge of economics, political science and other social sciences.

56. Central planning should aim at enabling communities to plan their own primary health care activities. It therefore has to provide them with a clear idea of the part they play in the national primary health care strategy and in the overall development process at community level. It has to guide them on how to work out, operate, evaluate and control their primary health care programmes; and it has to provide any essential information that is not available in the community.

57. Strengthened by this guidance and information, members of the community are better equipped to participate fully in the formulation of their primary health care programmes, by analysing their own health problems, taking decisions on priorities, making local adaptations of national solutions, and establishing their own community organization and support and control mechanisms. Wherever possible, those responsible for implementing programmes should participate actively in planning them from the earliest stages. In practice, steps have to be taken to ensure the continuity of the planning process, taking into account that responsibilities for planning and implementation may change hands from time to time.

58. Ideally, information concerning the primary health care programmes of all communities is fed back through the other levels of the health system to be used for the planning of support and referral at those levels, and for the consolidation of the nationwide programme. Constant interaction is therefore needed between the central levels, where policy is set, major resource allocations made, and standards and criteria established, and the intermediate and community levels, where detailed programmes are developed.

Planning and organization of primary health care in a community

59. Ways of planning and organizing primary health care in communities will vary with the type and size of community and with its pattern of social organization. Thus, solutions applicable to small villages may be vastly different from those appropriate for large urban communities. Nevertheless, certain features have to be taken into account that are common to all forms of community.

60. It is necessary to decide on the most suitable *mechanisms* for planning, operating and controlling the community primary health care programme. Local political, administrative and social patterns will help to determine these mechanisms. In all cases, it is necessary to reach agreement on responsibilities—for example, to decide who carries ultimate responsibility for the programme and whether the same individual, or committee as the case may be, is also responsible for its detailed planning and management. If a committee is elected, how should it be composed—of political or other community leaders, health workers or representatives of the public, and in what proportions? Will such a committee be given absolute powers, or will it be empowered only to make proposals, and if so to whom, or to which body representing the community as a whole? How will coordination with other sectors best be ensured—by including their representatives in the mechanism for planning and organizing primary health care, or by creating another community group consisting of representatives of all the sectors involved in development?

61. In determining *priorities*, what are the best ways of ensuring that the voice of the whole community is heard? And once priorities have been determined, are they to be given effect all at once or in stages? The answer to this last question will of course depend on the resources available; decisions have to be taken concerning the generation of local resources in cash and kind, and assessments made of the resources potentially available from the other levels of the health system and from central government. It is also necessary to decide who will deal with the other levels of the health system—for example, health workers at the technical level, or community leaders at the political level, or both.

62. Once priorities are decided on, decisions have to be taken concerning the *methods and techniques* to be employed. These have to be acceptable both to those who use them and to those on whom they are used. Also, an appropriate mechanism is required for taking these decisions, preferably including participants from the general public and from the health sector. Further decisions have to be taken on the composition and degree of skill of the health team providing primary health care. Should this be composed of health workers each providing the same range of service, or by a mixture of health workers each providing different kinds of service? Are there to be part-time or full-time health workers or a combination of both? What should be the conditions for their selection and by whom will they be selected? Should they be remunerated and, if so, how and on what scale? Will they have prospects for advancing in their career and how will this be organized and controlled? Should volunteers be mobilized?

63. What kind of basic *training* should the members of the health team receive and for how long? How will their continuing training be organized, who will organize it and who will provide it? Who will be appointed team leader? How will individuals and families be incorporated in the health team so that they become full partners in their own health development? How will they be educated in health matters and by whom?

64. When decisions have been taken on the methods to be employed for each of the components of primary health care, and on the types of health worker to apply these methods, it will be possible to decide on the *equipment and supplies* required, the essential drugs and vaccines, the system of maintaining equipment and the frequency of replenishing supplies. A balance will have to be reached between local considerations and national standards, taking into account local initiative and development on the one had, and the possibilities of organizing a national system of maintenance and supply on the other. Decisions also have to be taken on the *physical facilities* required, their location and size, and their design or adaptation from an existing structure.

65.   To control the implementation of the community programme, it is necessary to decide on the methods and mechanisms for social, managerial and technical guidance and *supervision*. Who will have overall responsibility within the primary health care facility? To whom will the person responsible report on progress and how often? To whom will this person turn with managerial, technical or social problems? To whom will the members of the community turn when they have similar problems?

66.   These are only some illustrations of the types of question that have to be answered in planning and operating a community primary health care programme. Whatever the solution, there is a need for clear-cut procedures that are known to the community as a whole and to the health workers and are followed by all concerned.

Coverage and accessibility

67.   Primary health care aims at providing the whole population with essential health care. *Population coverage* has often been expressed in terms of a numerical ratio between services for providing health care and the population to be served—for example, the number of hospital beds per unit of population, the number of doctors and nurses per unit of population or the number of people for whom a health centre has been established. Such ratios are often misleading. It is necessary to relate the specific components of health care being provided to those who require them—for example, to relate the provision of child care to the total number of children in the community, female as well as male, in order to make sure that such care is in fact available to all children. Even then, such ratios express the mere existence or availability of services and in no way show to what extent they have been used, let alone correctly used. To be used they have to be properly accessible.

68.   *Accessibility* implies the continuing and organized supply of care that is geographically, financially, culturally and functionnally within easy reach of the whole community. The care has to be ap-

propriate and adequate in content and in amount to satisfy the essential health needs of the people, and it has to be provided by methods acceptable to them.

69.   *Geographical accessibility* means that the distance, travel time and means of transportation are acceptable to the people. *Financial accessibility* means that whatever the methods of payment used, the services can be afforded by the community and the country. *Cultural accessibility* means that the technical and managerial methods used are in keeping with the cultural patterns of the community. *Functional accessibility* means that the right kind of care is available on a continuing basis to those who need it, whenever they need it, and that it is provided by the health team required for its proper delivery.

70.   The accessibility of primary health care has to be measured not only by its use at community level but also by the degree to which more complex problems can be solved, and people requiring more complex care treated, at the other levels of the health system. Primary health care that is fully and universally accessible is thus a means to ensure that the whole health system is used in a rational way.

71.   It is evident that accessibility will be defined in different ways in different societies and at different degrees of development of the same society. Each society at each stage will have to define criteria for measuring accessibility in the light of the factors mentioned above.

72.   An important factor for the success of primary health care is the use of appropriate health technology. The word "technology" means an association of methods, techniques and equipment which, together with the people using them, can contribute significantly to solving a health problem. "Appropriate" means that besides being scientifically sound the technology is also acceptable to those who apply it and to those for whom it is used. This implies that technology should be in keeping with the local culture. It must be capable of

Appropriate health technology

being adapted and further developed if necessary. In addition, it should preferably be easily understood and applied by community health workers, and in some instances even by individuals in the community; although different forms of technology are appropriate at different stage of development, their simplicity is always desirable. The most productive approach for ensuring that appropriate technology is available is to start with the problem and then to seek, or if necessary develop, a technology which is relevant to local conditions and resources.

73. Medicinal drugs are an important component of health technology. It is universally agreed that fewer drugs are necessary than the number at present on the market in most parts of the world. A model list of about 200 essential drugs is now available, prepared after international consultation.[1] The number of drugs needed for primary health care may be lower than 200, but this list can be used as a basis from which to select those drugs required in specific local circumstances. Drugs for use in the community should be simply and clearly labelled, carry clear instructions, and be safe for community health workers to use.

74. The identification or development of appropriate technology has to be considered when the national strategy for primary health care is being formulated. It is an advantage if the equipment and drugs selected can be manufactured locally at low cost. Also, the maintenance of equipment should preferably be within the capacity of local people and local facilities. Indigenous materials can often be used for small-scale manufacture of equipment within the country, renewable materials and sources of energy being preferably employed. If certain equipment and supplies cannot be produced and maintained locally, production facilities are required for whole districts or for the entire country, to ensure a degree of uniformity that will facilitate supply and maintenance.

---

[1] WHO Technical Report Series, No. 615, 1977 (*The selection of essential drugs:* report of a WHO Expert Committee).

75.   The principle that technology should be appropriate in the sense described above applies not only to primary health care in the community, but also to all the supportive levels, and especially to those closest to the community, such as health centres or district hospitals.

76.   It is part of national primary health care policy to insist on technology that is appropriate, to encourage its local development, to disseminate information about it and to promote its widespread use.

77.   People are the most important resource of any country, but all too often this resource remains untapped.   Primary health care, however, has to make full use of all available resources, and therefore has to mobilize the human potential of the entire community.   This is possible on condition that individuals and families accept greater responsibility for their health.   Their active interest and participation in solving their own health problems are not only a clear manifestation of social awareness and self-reliance but are also an important factor in ensuring the success of primary health care.   By their involvement, individuals become full members of the health team, whose joint action is essential to make the most of what primary health care has to offer.

Human resources

78.   In addition to community health workers and members of the community themselves, the health team will include personnel in establishments at the supporting levels.   The composition of the team will vary according to the varying needs of groups of the population, for if primary health care is the hub of the health system, people in need are the hub of primary health care.

79.   At the first level of contact between individuals and the health care system, primary health care is provided by community health workers acting as a team.   The *types of health worker* will vary by country and community according to needs and the resources available for satisfying them.   Thus, they may include in different societies

Community health workers

people with limited education who have been given elementary training in health care, "barefoot doctors", medical assistants, practical and professionally trained nurses, feldschers, and general medical practitioners, as well as traditional practitioners.

80.   For many developing countries, the most realistic solution for attaining total population coverage with essential health care is to employ *community health workers* who can be trained in a short time to perform specific tasks.   They may be required to carry out a wide range of health care activities, or, alternatively, their functions may be restricted to certain aspects of health care, the total range being provided by a team of health workers, each performing a specific group of tasks.   In many societies, it is advantageous if these health workers come from the community in which they live and are chosen by it, so that they have its support.   Where they come from other communities, it is important that they become socially attuned to the way of life of the community they are to serve.   They are given a short, simple training to prepare them to perform the kinds of activity that respond to the expressed needs of the community;   this training can gradually be extended to cover additional tasks as required.   Since much of their time will be devoted to education, they must be adequately prepared for this activity.

81.   Community health workers have to be trained and retrained so that they can play a progressively more important role in providing primary health care.   Their *training and retraining* should be based on a clear definition of the problems involved, the tasks to be performed, and the methods, techniques and equipment to be used.   Instruction is best carried out in accordance with modern teaching/learning methods, and as far as possible should take place in the vicinity of the communities to be served.   The length of training is best determined in the light of the educational aims and the results of preliminary testing of individuals, since training has to be adapted to their degree of literacy. Other considerations are the need to prepare them to work in a team and the need to provide them with an understanding of the relation-

ships between their work and that of representatives of other sectors also concerned, since cooperation among them all can have a marked effect on community development. Continuing training programmes have to take account of the need for management capabilities and supervisory responsibilities. In parallel with continuing education, consideration has to be given to the careers of community health workers and their opportunities for advancement.

82. Traditional medical practitioners and birth attendants are found in most societies. They are often part of the local community, culture and traditions, and continue to have high social standing in many places, exerting considerable influence on local health practices. With the support of the formal health system, these indigenous practitioners can become important allies in organizing efforts to improve the health of the community. Some communities may select them as community health workers. It is therefore well worth while exploring the possibilities of engaging them in primary health care and of training them accordingly.

Traditional medical practitioners

83. When more complicated care, or advice on complex problems, are needed, the community health worker should be able to turn for help to more highly trained staff. The categories of such staff used at the different levels of the health system will vary according to the resources in each country. [Whatever the arrangement, their work is given a new orientation by the need to support and strengthen primary health care.] The responsibilities of more highly trained staff are also increased, since they have to apply their technical skills to solve health problems determined in the light of social needs, to guide, teach and supervise community health workers, and to educate communities on all matters pertaining to their health. They are therefore given social and educational functions in addition to their technical functions, and [if they accept this challenge they can become leaders in health.] Problem

Professional health workers

Family members   84.   Family members are often the main providers of health care. In most societies, *women* play an important role in promoting health, particularly in view of their central position in the family; this means that they can contribute significantly to primary health care, especially in ensuring the application of preventive measures. Women's organizations in the community can be encouraged to discuss such questions as nutrition, child care, sanitation and family planning. In addition to being important for health promotion, these organizations can stimulate the interest of women in other activities likely to enhance the quality of community life.

85.   Other family members also make major contributions. *Young people* can be educated to have a good understanding of what health means, how to achieve it, and how it contributes to development. They can be very effective in taking these messages to their homes and interpreting new ideas to their families, as well as being useful in practical work, for example in the fields of first aid and basic sanitation. *Old people* can also be given many tasks which contribute to the health of the community and which at the same time improve their own health by giving them a social purpose. It is important to encourage *men*, too, to take a greater interest in health, and to help them realize that they can contribute by shaping the community health system, as well as by taking part in practical undertakings. Such participation also has the incidental benefit of providing men with a better understanding of what community health development really means.

Referral system   86.   As explained in the section on the place of primary health care in the health system, primary health care activities in the community are supported by successive levels of referral facilities. These engage more highly trained staff capable of dealing with a progressively wider range of specialized health interventions that require more sophisticated technology than can be provided at the community level.

87.   Additional thought will have to be given to referral facilities, and especially to the establishments that constitute the link next to

primary health care in the health system chain. In particular, there is a need to review the functions, staffing, planning, design, equipment, organization and management of health centres and district hospitals, in order to prepare them for their wider function in support of primary health care. These establishments will have to adopt a new role in response to the needs of primary health care. Since the problems arising will be on a wider scale than the clinical problems of the seriously ill, the range of services provided will have to be correspondingly wider. They will include the continuing training, guidance and supervision of community health workers as well as the education of the community in health matters. These establishments will have to provide guidance on sanitary measures and to disseminate information on disease control methods that are suitable locally. They will have to provide logistic support in supplying pesticides, drugs, and sanitary and medical equipment. They will of course continue to provide specialized clinical outpatient and inpatient care. Their responsibilities will also involve liaison and intervention with other sectors involved in social and economic development at the administrative level concerned. Such extramural involvement is essential to create confidence in the whole system and to avoid overloading the referral institutions with people who do not need their facilities but could be looked after in the community by primary health care.

88. Referral for more specialized care is best organized according to procedures clearly laid down for each level. This arrangement ensures that each part of the referral chain performs first and foremost the functions for which it is intended, bearing in mind that as far as possible health interventions should take place at community level.

89. The transportation of patients to and from referral services has to be properly organized, making the most of available facilities. Sometimes, unnecessary transportation can be avoided if advice can be given over a communication link by whatever means exist or can be provided at low cost.

90. It should be emphasized that referral is a two-way process and that the retention of patients in a referral institution should be as brief as possible. As soon as their recovery can be maintained by simpler means, they are best returned to the community, accompanied by clear information on the clinical findings and care provided, as well as guidance concerning the further care required.

Logistics of supply
91. Once the decision has been taken to adopt primary health care, it is necessary to make supplies available to communities on a priority basis. The process of supply begins with decisions on the components to be included in the community's primary health care programme, and the technologies to be employed for each of these components. Supplies are then planned for, ordered and delivered in accordance with the requirements for those technologies. It is useful to have available standard lists of drugs and equipment, reduced to the minimum, that take into account the epidemiological situation as well as the resources available. While certain basic items may be the same for a large number of communities, there may also have to be adjustments to take account of local variations, such as seasonal fluctuations in the incidence of certain diseases. Supply therefore has to be planned as an integral part of the formulation of primary health programmes at the different levels.

92. The logistics of supply include planning and budgeting for the supplies required, procurement or manufacture, storage, distribution and control. Supplies of the right quality and quantity have to be delivered to primary health care facilities at the right time to make it possible to provide services on a continuing basis. The time needed to carry out the various steps in the purchase and distribution of different kinds of supplies has to be taken into account, and administrative procedures have to be applied that will ensure the continuity of supply.

93. In developing a supply system, consideration has to be given both to cost and to national and local production as part of overall development. For example, it may be cheaper to buy certain items

abroad, but economically more productive in the long run to produce them within the country. This principle may apply also to the alternatives of national purchasing and local production.

94. The physical facilities required for primary health care may be very simple but they must be very clean. They need not necessarily be built specially for the purpose, nor used exclusively for health care. In many communities there already exists some building which can be easily adapted and used for both health and other community activities. Frequently this is a successful combination, since people become accustomed to congregating at this central point and enjoy meeting one another there.

Physical facilities

95. If a building does have to be specially built, the members of the community can often do this with their own labour and materials. It can be a place that remains under their care and responsibility and where they feel at home. An important point to be remembered is that a large number of people will probably use the building, which should therefore have a spacious waiting area, either inside or under cover outside, with toilets.

96. In many countries physical facilities are particularly lacking at the first referral level, that is, at the level next in line from primary health care. Here, more substantial buildings and equipment are required. It is a matter of priority to strengthen this often weak link in the chain with adequate investments, so that these facilities can be used to support primary health care in the way outlined in paragraphs 86—90.

97. To make sure that the principles of primary health care are translated into practice, a national managerial process is required. This includes planning, programming, budgeting, financing, control of implementation, evaluation, research, replanning if necessary, and in-

National managerial process

formation support for all these activities. Reference has already been made to broad planning at the central level whereby decisions are taken which foster the development of primary health care within communities and responsibility is delegated both to them, for planning and operating their programmes, and to the other levels of the health system for planning and operating their support to primary health care.

98.   An essential decision that has to be taken at an early stage at the central level is to give priority to primary health care both at the community level and at the supporting levels. This fundamental decision then has to be translated into budgetary terms to make it possible to implement it.

Budgeting   99.   Budgeting at the central level is a key step because it estimates required resources and allocates those available in such a way as to transform an intention into concrete realization of the programme at the various levels of the health system. Thus, budgeting has to ensure the preferential allocation of resources to primary health care, starting from communities and progressing through the other levels. It consists basically of the allocation to communities and to supporting services of financial ceilings which are to be used for the particular purposes defined in the primary health care programme. It should be emphasized, however, that budgeting of this kind does not need to be built up from a precise addition of items requested by each community. Much time and effort can be saved by the allocation of resources according to an overall estimate of needs, based on programme objectives and common approaches for attaining them, and using standard costs.

Decentralization   100.   Budgetary allocations need to be accompanied by simultaneous delegation of responsibility and authority. Thus, communities are each given a certain financial ceiling together with the responsibility and the authority to use that money, in addition to their own resources in cash and kind, in order to develop primary health care in accordance with the programme they have worked out. At the other levels also, funds are allocated and responsibility and authority are given for the specific purpose of supporting primary health care in the communities they are serving. This approach helps to ensure that the programme is carried out by earmarking funds to be used only for the purpose of primary health care and support to it.

101. Primary health care, with its supporting services, has to be **Control** controlled in the sense of ensuring as far as possible that it is functioning in accordance with the national policy and strategy.

102. The community itself to a large extent provides managerial control for primary health care through various mechanisms designed to make sure that the measures decided on are being applied and that activities are being carried out as planned. Any deviations can be reported on quickly and corrected at the source, or alternatively endorsed if they seem better than the measures and activities originally envisaged.

103. Control of a technical nature comes from the more specialized levels of the health system, through guidance, education and provision of the right kind of information, accompanied by readiness to deal with more complex problems.

104. Control of primary health care therefore implies supervision, but with the double connotation of managerial control by the community combined with technical guidance and support from the other levels of the health system, provided within a true process of education.

105. In order to ensure that primary health care is functioning **Evaluation** properly and that the lessons learned in the course of its operation are used to improve the programme, a process of evaluation has to be built in. Evaluation is carried out by those providing the services, those

using them, and those responsible for managerial and technical control at the different levels of the health system. Thus, a dialogue is created among all involved, based on their respective assessments but always with a view to improving primary health care. Making evaluation an integral part of the programme also helps to keep its costs as low as possible.

106.   Evaluation has several components. It is first necessary to review the *relevance* of the activities being carried out in terms of their consistency with the social philosophy of the programme. Then, an analysis is made of *progress* in carrying out activities as planned in order to facilitate operational control. Assessment of the *efficiency* with which the programme is being carried out aims at improving implementation by comparing the results obtained with the efforts expended, the latter being expressed in terms of people, time, money and health technologies. It includes the measure of the extent to which facilities are actually being used. Review of the *effectiveness* of the programme aims at measuring the extent to which it appears to be reducing the severity of specific conditions or improving the health situation in the community. It could also include an assessment of the degree of community participation in the programme and satisfaction with it. *Impact* is an expression of the effect the programme is having on the overall socioeconomic development of the community.

107.   There is a need for certain indicators to measure change, and various criteria against which actions can be compared. For example, indicators have to be defined to assess any increase in the coverage of the community with safe drinking-water, or improvement in the health status of children. As another example, since one of the aims of primary health care is universal accessibility of essential health care, criteria have to be developed to assess accessibility, based for example on the factors mentioned in paragraphs 68—71. When formal indicators and criteria are not available, asking simple questions can often be useful, such as "Are the methods being used really acceptable to children?" or "Do all people in fact have access to the facilities and are they using them properly?".

108. In order to plan and manage primary health care the right **Information** kind of information is essential, but the collection of information has to be kept to the minimum required. It is important to identify only that relevant information which is going to be used in the community or the referral service. In many instances it is more important to start with qualitative information on the health and demographic situation than attempt to gather precise quantified data. Quantitative precision can be built up in the course of time. Every level of the health system has its own information requirements concerning primary health care, and the same information may call for a different degree of elaboration and aggregation at each level.

109. To be of practical use, the reporting of information from one level to another has to be two-way, only that information which is actually required by the other level being transmitted. Usually this information will be of two types: information in response to which immediate action is required, and information on which to base more general inferences, evaluation and subsequent modification of programmes as required.

110. Any information-gathering and analysis required should be an integral part of primary health care activities and their supporting services; they should not be carried out separately. They need to be included in plans from the beginning, and information should be gathered or transmitted only for the two purposes just mentioned, and be restricted to the minimum.

111. Enough is already known about primary health care for it to **Research** be put into practice immediately. However, much still needs to be learned about its application under local conditions, and during its operation, control and evaluation problems will arise which require research. These may be related to such questions as the organization of primary health care within communities and of supporting services; the mobilization of community support and participation; the best ways

of applying technology available or the development of new technologies as required; the planning for and training of community health workers, their supervision, their remuneration and their career structure; and methods of financing primary health care. Whatever the substance of the research, building it into the programme from the outset makes it a practical way of promoting continuous improvement.

Financing   112.   In paragraph 99 mention was made of the essential decision to give preferential allocation of resources to primary health care and its supporting system. Account has to be taken of any community participation in financing community services, but in most countries financing is likely to be a combined community and government effort, with the government in the final analysis having to ensure that it is adequate for the programme agreed on. Finance for health care may come from government taxation, or from a social security system, with contributions from individuals or employers or both, and it may also come from philanthropic sources or through payment by individuals. However, for developing countries to rely solely on methods of financing health care that are current in more affluent countries will be as unwise as to rely on the technology practised in those countries. Thus, the coverage of primary health care costs through national taxation may be quite impracticable and totally inadequate in predominantly agricultural societies. Also, the classical social security systems applied in some of the industrial countries may, in developing countries, tend to favour very limited population groups and thus lead to discrimination against the majority of the population. Individual payment on a fee-for-service basis is certainly not a solution that can be widely applied. In addition, such social security and private methods of payment may be totally inapplicable to some vital components of primary health care that are not concerned with direct service to individuals, such as the provision of potable water, the protection of houses against insects and rodents, or health education in all its aspects.

113.   It is therefore necessary to keep an open mind on methods of financing primary health care. Every country has to evolve its own

methods, based on its own circumstances and judgement, analysing the experiences of others in the light of its own political, social and economic context, experimenting as necessary and informing others of the results of its experimentation. For example, in many countries even slight increases in the productivity of large sections of society would change their patterns of consumption and make them capable of shouldering part of the financial burden of health development. In some societies, if people were properly motivated and trained, greater use could be made of voluntary service for various health actions, including the development of local water supplies or part-time service in the delivery of health care.

114. Where all health services are provided by the government it is possible to control not only the organization and budgeting of primary health care but its financing too. Where the health system is composed of multiple agencies, it is important to coordinate the resources as well as the efforts of all of them and to induce them to lend their weight to primary health care and its supporting structures.

115. National nongovernmental organizations should be encouraged to finance primary health care and the services that support it. The external financial support required by many countries should be channelled in the same direction. External financing may take the form of loans and grants from bilateral and multilateral sources, and countries must weigh the advantages and disavantages of accepting financial support from these sources. In addition to providing funds for immediate use, external financing can stimulate the appropriation of additional national funds, thus facilitating the introduction of national programmes and speeding up countrywide coverage. However, care has to be taken that external financing does not replace national efforts, which are needed to ensure the continuity and further development of primary health care.

4. National Strategies and International Support

National and international commitment

116. Firm national commitment to primary health care is vital, but it must be clear what this commitment entails. It has been shown that primary health care has a great variety of implications and consequences that go far beyond technical considerations. National strategies are therefore required that take into account all political, social and economic as well as technical factors, and that help to overcome obstacles of any nature. Such strategies should aim at creating a climate that will make primary health care objectives, targets and activities feasible. International political support is also important in order to foster this climate and to help individual governments to overcome their difficulties.

National strategies

117. Reference has already been made in chapter 3 to the process of translating policies for primary health care into practical programmes and to the need for a specific strategy for formulation and implementation. It is important that programme formulation be carried out on a countrywide basis. The national programme may begin in selected parts of the country, provided that all are covered as soon as possible. It may also start with only a limited number of the components of primary health care, provided that the others are added in the course of time. The essential feature is that it should be extended progressively, in both geographical coverage and content, until it covers all the population with all essential components. The national strategy will include the referral systems already mentioned, and support from relevant components of other sectors such as education, transport, agriculture and sectors dealing with the environment.

118.   The success of the strategy will depend in the final analysis on whether it reflects the full commitment of the government as a whole.   Commitment is important to develop and launch the strategy and to maintain its momentum.   Such political will is essential to make sure that preferential allocation of resources is being given to primary health care, that communities are being supported in planning their own health care programmes, and that all the sectors involved are coordinating their efforts.   However, if it is not possible to implement strategies in accordance with a strictly rational process of decision-making, a pragmatic approach may have to be adopted in order to seize every opportunity to introduce primary health care whenever and wherever possible.

119.   The overall objective for which the strategy is intended is to provide essential health care to all the population.   It is necessary to define any intermediate stages required in order to reach this ultimate goal.   The following are some of the most important steps that have to be taken to devise and implement the strategy.

Basis for a strategy

120.   It is necessary to define the *communities* in need of such care, to decide on their grouping for the purposes of support and referral, and to make sure that the other levels of the health system are properly geared to provide the support required.

121.   There is a need to ensure that central planning really does promote *decentralized community planning*, that the health budget gives priority allocation of *funds* to primary health care and its support mechanisms, and that *responsibility and authority* are delegated. Equally, it is important to ensure proper *coordination* at the community, intermediate and central levels with all other sectors involved.

122.   *Information* has to be made available on technologies that can be used and the best ways of applying them. A *supply system* has to be organized, *guidelines* have to be provided for the physical facilities, equipment and supplies required. Appropriate *training* has to be

ensured. *Research* capacities have to be developed, for instance to improve knowledge which can actually be applied in the programme, or to ensure the application of the programme in various social and cultural contexts.

123.   Finally, it is important to develop mechanisms for *technical cooperation among developing countries*, both to provide and to absorb experience and to ensure that external funds are channelled into primary health care and properly allocated.

Mobilizing public opinion   124.   One of the fundamental principles of primary health care is the participation of the community at all stages. For communities to be intelligently involved, they need to have easy access to the right kind of information concerning their health situation and how they themselves can help to improve it. Of particular importance is a clear explanation of the technologies available, their advantages and disadvantages, their successes and failures, their possible adverse effects, and their costs. The information given should be neither oversophisticated nor condescending but should be in a language people can understand. Newspapers, magazines, radio, television, films, plays, posters, community notice-boards and any other means available can be used to secure people's enthusiasm and their willingness to get primary health care going in the right direction.

Legislation   125.   In some countries, legislation will be required to facilitate the development of primary health care and the implementation of its strategy. Thus, there might be a need for new legislation or the revision of existing legislation, to permit communities to plan, manage and control primary health care and to allow various types of health workers to perform duties hitherto carried out exclusively by health professionals. On the other hand, there often exist laws which are not applied but which, as they stand, might be used to facilitate the development of primary health care.

126. Full development of the primary health care programme and achievement of its fundamental purposes is a long-term process, and the strategy must take this into account. New knowledge gained from national and international activities as well as from research must be incorporated. It is therefore wise for each country to create mechanisms that will help it to absorb information on experience of primary health care. The strategy will need to be continually adjusted in the light of this information, the country's own experience, and the social changes that are bound to take place in the course of time.

A long-term approach

127. Primary health care involves a major rethinking of ways of delivering health care. To make the community the focal point of the whole health system, to look for the relevant technology that countries and communities can accept and afford, and to aim at the universal accessibility of health care is in many ways revolutionary. Primary health care will be more acceptable and easier to implement for all countries if they realize that others are successfully using this approach. For this reason, international political, moral, technical and financial support are important.

International support

128. The type of external support needed must be very carefully identified and coordinated by the receiving country itself. The government has the responsibility for defining areas for which external support is needed. This is a manifestation of the principle of national self-reliance in health matters. Interagency coordination of international support must always be based on this principle.

129. While the primary health care approach itself is universal, there is no universal recipe for primary health care programmes, each one being a national endeavour specific to the country's situation. What succeeds in one country cannot necessarily be transplanted and have the same results elsewhere. Nevertheless, certain factors do emerge from national experiences which can serve as a guide to others, so international cooperation in this area is likely to be fruitful.

Technical cooperation and technical cooperation among developing countries

130.   Mutual support of countries for primary health care programmes will consist mainly in the sharing of expertise and training facilities, the development of appropriate technology and the exchange of information and experience, using national institutions.   While the role of the developed countries in providing financial and technical support will continue to be extremely helpful, there is particular scope in primary health care for the application of technical cooperation among developing countries.   The role of international health agencies will be mainly to promote and support this kind of technical cooperation among developing countries, as well as between industrialized and developing countries.   This promotive and supportive role too can best be executed through the proper use of national institutions.

Financial support

131.   Primary health care as envisaged above, especially during its evolutionary phase and particularly in developing countries, requires considerable financial resources.   This support for primary health care has to be very carefully channelled.   In the past, most financial support has gone to highly sophisticated and specialized medical services for small privileged groups.   It is now necessary to reverse this trend and focus the support on primary health care.   As an expression of the international political commitment and support mentioned in paragraphs 116 and 128, the affluent countries would do well to increase substantially the transfer of funds to the developing countries for primary health care.   Flexibility in the use of these funds is important so that receiving countries can allocate them where they are most required. Requirements for care in the community are self-evident.   However, because of the need to reorient the health system so that it supports primary health care, and to facilitate the process of referral to the appropriate form of specialized health care, it should also be possible to use these external financial resources for health centres and district hospitals on condition that they are fully supporting primary health care.   Such politically motivated support, coupled with the additional resources that the developing countries themselves can generate within the context of the New International Economic Order, will add a genuine developmental potential to international collaboration.

132. National and international nongovernmental organizations can make a very useful contribution to primary health care programmes, precisely because they work within the community. They have the same responsibility as international governmental organizations in the sense that they provide technical and financial support to countries and would do well to ensure that these are channelled into the promotion of primary health care and its supporting system.

Non-governmental organizations

133. In conclusion, international commitment to primary health care should be oriented to support national primary health care programmes by creating a positive climate of opinion; by facilitating the exchange of expertise, technology and information through technical cooperation among developing countries and between industrialized and developing countries; and by encouraging proper orientation of financial resources. However, all international agencies, nongovernmental organizations and countries providing support have to be aware that the purpose of their efforts is in the long run to enable countries themselves to apply primary health care as part of their overall development and in the spirit of self-reliance.

Respect for national self-reliance